Curcumin

The 21st Century Cure

Jan McBarron, M.D., N.D.

An Imprint of Take Charge Books
Brevard, NC

The purpose of this book is to educate. It is not intended to serve as a replacement for professional medical advice. Any use of the information in this book is at the reader's discretion. This book is sold with the understanding that neither the publisher nor the author has any liability or responsibility for any injury caused or alleged to be caused directly or indirectly by the information contained in this book. While every effort has been made to ensure its accuracy, the book's contents should not be construed as medical advice. To obtain medical advice on your individual health needs, please consult a qualified health care practitioner.

Library of Congress Cataloging-in Publication Data is on file with the Library of Congress.

ISBN: 978-0-9883866-3-1

Editor: Kathleen Barnes
Cover and interior design: Gary A. Rosenberg

Printed in the United States of America

10   9   8   7   6   5   4   3   2   1

Contents

CHAPTER I

What Is Curcumin and How Does It Work?

AN ASIAN SECRET FOR LONGEVITY

What if I told you there is a common spice that can give you the gift of a long and healthy life? How about an extract of this familiar spice that can prevent and even cure heart disease, cancer, diabetes, Alzheimer's disease, depression, joint pain and more?

Maybe you would think it's just a bunch of hype, but I can assure you there is voluminous scientific research that warrants placing curcumin at the pinnacle of all healing herbs.

If you love curry, you'll be familiar with turmeric, a popular vividly-colored spice. Inside turmeric is a compound called curcumin, which is found in its rhizome (the stem of the plant found underground). Curcumin is responsible for the golden orange color of turmeric, and is perhaps the most powerful botanical medicine in the world today. *However, there is very little curcumin in the spice turmeric.* If you've seen cheap turmeric supplements on the market understand that they only contain 2 to 5% curcumin, which may or may not be usable by your body, and they're not likely to have any effectiveness in terms of prevention or treatment for the diseases we're talking about. Curcumin is *many times* more powerful than turmeric.

For centuries, curcumin has given the gift of long life and robust health to the people of India, for whom various types of curries—always made with turmeric—are a dietary staple. Curcumin is an important ingredient in the Ayurvedic medicine tradition and a vital part of Traditional Chinese Medicine. Now I can say without equivocation that it is the cure-all of the 21st century, backed by voluminous research that credits its healing powers to its exceptional antioxidant and anti-inflammatory properties.

Botanically known as *Curcuma longa*, the turmeric rhizome is a member of the antioxidant-rich ginger family. You might be understandably skeptical when you hear that this humble Indian spice can prevent, treat and cure a wide variety of serious diseases. These include everything from heart attacks to a dozen types of cancer, the pain of all types of arthritis and even "incurable" diseases like diabetes and Alzheimer's. Curcumin also soothes depression and the agony of a variety of digestive disorders, including Crohn's disease, inflammatory bowel disease and irritable bowel syndrome.

In this book, I'll address your skepticism with an in-depth examination of each of these conditions and the research supporting curcumin's role in prevention, treatment and cure.

CURCUMIN: THE TRIPLE WHAMMY AGAINST CHRONIC DISEASE

Curcumin has proven antioxidant, anti-inflammatory and anticancer properties. This takes in most, if not all, of the chronic diseases of aging known to modern science.

Think about rust on the bumper of a car. Rust is caused by oxidation or damaging oxygen molecules that corrode and eventually destroy the structure of metal.

Those same corrosive oxygen molecules (sometimes called free radicals) are found inside the human body, and while they are part of the aging process, they are an unpleasant part of it because they contribute to the deterioration of cells. When these "rusty" cells reproduce, each generation is just a little different from the last and a little bit less able to perform its function properly. That, in a nutshell, is how and why we age.

The oxidative aging process is escalated by environmental factors:

- Polluted air and water

- Plastics and other toxic materials that contaminate nearly everything we touch, eat and drink

- Pesticides and other poisons and hormones in our food and even in our clothing

- Processed foods, smoking, obesity, lack of exercise and other unhealthy lifestyle choices

OXIDATION AND INFLAMMATION CAUSE DISEASE

So, what happens when we get "rust" or oxidative damage in our cells? Our brain cells begin to deteriorate, so memory becomes

A handful of devastating diseases of aging are all partially or totally caused by oxidation:

❖ Heart disease ❖ Osteoarthritis

❖ Cancer ❖ Alzheimer's disease

❖ Diabetes ❖ Dementia

fuzzy; our hearts don't beat as efficiently as they once did; our arteries become clogged; our blood sugars spike and cellular division is thrown so far out of whack that our cells begin to divide wildly, creating cancers that can kill us.

This oxidative stress can also cause brain chemistry to malfunction, resulting in depression, one of the most common and debilitating diseases of modern times.

Worst of all, these nasty free radical oxygen molecules cause inflammation, with obvious results if you think of arthritis, joint pain and other forms of chronic pain, but less obvious ones as underlying causes of all of the degenerative diseases already mentioned.

In addition, obesity and inflammation go hand-in-hand. Most likely, obesity causes inflammation, although the scientific community isn't quite convinced yet. More than 40% of all Americans are obese. When we add in those 30% who are overweight but not yet obese, we find that excess weight plagues 70% of all American adults. That makes the inflammation associated with obesity a serious contributing factor in all of the diseases of aging.

THE GOLDEN KNIGHT

Like a golden knight on a palomino charger, curcumin rides to the rescue!

Curcumin is by far the most powerful antioxidant known to science, hundreds of times more powerful than blueberries, which have substantial antioxidant capabilities themselves.

On the ORAC (Oxygen Radical Absorbance Capacity) scale that rates the antioxidant power of foods, only BCM-95® Curcumin rates over 1.5 million per 100 grams, while antioxidant-rich blueberries have only a 6,000 ORAC rating per 100 grams! This means that just one high-quality curcumin capsule delivers more than 25 times the antioxidants as the same amount of blueberries.

Curcumin literally scrubs the oxidative "rust" from your cells, preventing serious disease and reversing diseases you may already have. It helps stop cell deterioration and restores the cellular genetic codes to youthful levels, ensuring those cells will reproduce more like they did when you were young.

More important, from the viewpoint of damaged cell division found in cancer, curcumin also tells these cells to die when their time comes, as ordained by nature, which stops tumor growth.

And that wonderful yellow curcumin stops inflammation and all of its obvious and not-so-obvious damaging effects, relieving inflammatory problems like arthritis and joint pain and eliminating the building blocks for heart disease, diabetes and other diseases that have a foundation in chronic inflammation.

In addition, curcumin has a unique ability to cross the blood-brain barrier, a membrane that protects the brain from invaders like bacterial infections and keeps out most other substances as well, including those that might be helpful. This gives curcumin the ability to deliver its antioxidants and anti-inflammatories directly to the brain, which is particularly helpful in cases of dementia and depression.

In the case of cancer, cutting-edge research shows curcumin has a variety of ways of stopping abnormal cell growth, including an ability to affect cell division on the genetic level.

If that's not enough, studies also show that curcumin protects the liver and kidneys.

Curcumin has been compared to pharmaceutical drugs for the treatment of a wide variety of diseases, and it has come out on top in every case.

ANOTHER TRIPLE WHAMMY AGAINST INFLAMMATION

Inflammation is a factor in 80 to 90% of all disease, according to curcumin researcher Ajay Goel, Ph.D., director of Epigenetics and Cancer Prevention at Baylor University Medical Center in Dallas. What's not to love?

"Curcumin demonstrates superior antioxidant and anti-inflammatory effects and provides liver- and heart-protective benefits as well. It is a potent antibacterial, antifungal, antiviral, anti-allergenic and has antitumor and anti-cancer properties," says Dr. Goel.

By knocking out viruses, bacteria and fungi, curcumin offers the powerful possibility that we can use it to treat everything from colds and flu to pneumonia or even to help with something as serious as AIDS or cancer, effectively and without dangerous side effects.

ALL CURCUMIN IS NOT CREATED EQUAL

Unless you are willing to eat curry three times a day, you probably can't eat enough turmeric or curcumin to make much of a difference to your health. That's because in its most common form, curcumin is not very absorbable or bioavailable to the human body.

Fortunately, at least one company has found a way to make curcumin highly absorbable. In Chapter 10, you'll find more on Curamin® and CuraMed®, supplements containing BCM-95®, the highly absorbable form of curcumin that has been well-researched to produce the protective and curative results in scientific studies.

Launched in the U.S. market by EuroPharma Inc. under the *Terry Naturally* brand name, the amazing thing about BCM-95® is that it takes curcumin—a nutrient that is notoriously difficult to absorb—and makes it ready for the body to use. In fact, BCM-95® is up to ten times more absorbable (and retained in the bloodstream longer at more medicinal levels) than standard 95% curcumin extracts.

CHAPTER 2

Curcumin and Heart Disease

Since heart disease is the #1 killer in the Western world, any nutrient, like curcumin, that helps protect your heart and arteries and even reverses heart disease should be most welcome.

Curcumin's heart-protective effects become even more important when we add diabetes to the mix. Heart disease is the most common complication of diabetes, and the number of newly diagnosed diabetics is increasing dramatically every year, with nearly 2 million new cases reported among U.S. adults in 2010.

KEEP ARTERIES CLEAR

Clogged arteries raise the risk of heart attack and stroke. Fatty deposits (called plaque) cause arteries to narrow, reduce blood flow, make your heart work harder to move blood through the circulatory system and harden the arteries. In time, cholesterol buildup can completely block an artery and cause a heart attack or stroke.

Curcumin raises the levels of HDL or "good" cholesterol that helps move fats out of the cells, including the cells in the arteries. It also reduces the stickiness of blood cells, preventing clots.

With curcumin, cholesterol improvement can happen fast: An Indian study showed that human volunteers who took 500 milligrams a day for just a week increased their good (HDL) cholesterol by 29%.

In addition, inflammation is a foundational cause of cardio-vascular disease and there is abundant evidence that curcumin is one of the most potent anti-inflammatory substances known to science. Therefore, it stands to reason that reduction of inflammation also reduces the risk of heart disease and stroke. Other studies suggest that curcumin may actually change the messages sent by genes that signal the body to build up those fatty deposits in the arteries.

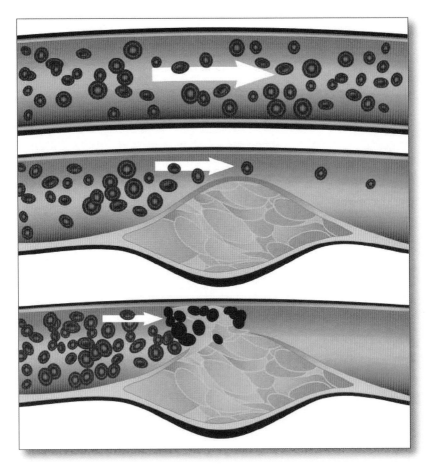

Image of arteries shows normal flow (top), constricted flow (center) and blocked artery (bottom).

REDUCE HOMOCYSTEINE AND CRP LEVELS

Homocysteine is an amino acid naturally present in the human body. When homocysteine starts to build up in the bloodstream, it increases the hardening and narrowing of the arteries, may cause blood clotting, raises your risk of heart disease and can be predictive of a heart attack, stroke and possibly Alzheimer's disease.

CRP (C-Reactive Protein) is a body signal of inflammation. It damages the arterial walls, resulting in hardening of the arteries and blood clotting. Curcumin helps to relax those arterial wall cells, reduces the hardening of the arteries and allows the blood to flow more freely, dissolving clots and preventing and even reversing plaque buildup.

REVERSE HEART FAILURE

Congestive heart failure occurs when the heart can no longer pump enough blood to the rest of the body. It is usually a slow process that gets worse over time. As the heart muscle loses its ability to pump oxygen-rich blood throughout the body, it causes fluid buildup in the lungs, liver, gastrointestinal tract, arms and legs. This lack of oxygen damages vital organs, eventually causing death.

Curcumin prevents the creation of scar tissue in the heart muscle and helps failing hearts return to their normal pumping capacity, according to breakthrough Canadian research published in 2008. Scientists at the Canadian Institutes of Health Research discovered that curcumin acts directly on the DNA of heart cells, preventing them from unraveling under physical stress. Curcumin was shown to switch off the "unraveling switch" in the heart cell DNA that keeps scar tissue from developing.

In the February 2008 edition of the *Journal of Clinical Investigation,* researchers at the Peter Munk Cardiac Centre of the Toronto General Hospital reported that curcumin may dramatically reduce the chance of developing heart failure.

"When the herb is given orally, it can actually prevent and reverse hypertrophy, restore heart function and reduce scar formation," researchers wrote.

PREVENT STROKE AND STOP STROKE DAMAGE

Strokes have two major causes. The most common is a blood clot that travels to the brain and the second is a ruptured blood vessel in the brain. As we learned earlier in this chapter, the buildup of cholesterol, elevated homocysteine and CRP levels and even congestive heart failure are risk factors for stroke as well as heart attack. Since stroke is a cardiovascular disease, a stroke is a "brain attack," if you will, similar to a heart attack. We already know that curcumin has powerful preventive and healing properties for all of these conditions.

Strokes almost inevitably damage brain cells. But exciting new research shows that curcumin, given intravenously, can minimize brain damage while a stroke is in progress because it can cross the blood-brain barrier, protecting the mechanisms that help regenerate brain cells. This is effective if it is administered in an emergency room within three hours of a stroke.

SUPER ANTIOXIDANT

Curcumin's antioxidant properties are one of its most potent weapons against all of the diseases commonly linked with the aging process, most notably cardiovascular disease. I like to think of antioxidants as "rust removers" of the body because they literally remove the "rust" or the foundational causes of the diseases of aging connected to excessive free-radical oxygen molecules.

Cholesterol or even excessive cholesterol in itself does not clog arteries. It is the oxidized cholesterol that clogs arteries, restricts blood flow to vital organs and eventually breaks away to cause heart attacks and strokes.

By preventing this oxidation in the first place, curcumin's antioxidant properties keep the arteries clear of that potentially fatal oxidized cholesterol or plaque.

CONCLUSION

Curcumin's abilities to protect your heart, brain and cardiovascular system are beyond impressive. Consider the drugs commonly used to treat the heart conditions discussed in this chapter. The statin drugs alone (Lipitor, Crestor and their cousins) carry with them huge health risks from side effects, including causing death from sudden heart failure.

It only makes sense to use substances that are effective as well as harmless.

Curcumin is natural and safe. Only rarely do people taking curcumin get mild stomach upset at dosages of 10 grams per day or more. What's more, even the highest quality products are very affordable. Who could ask for more?

CHAPTER 3

Curcumin and Cancer

Cancer arouses more fear in the human heart than any other disease. The dread is well placed, even though cancer is not the #1 killer in the Western world.

Every year, more than 1.5 million people are diagnosed with cancer, not including skin cancers, which are by far the most common cancers. Skin cancers afflict 2 million more people every year.

Each year, 569,000 of us will die of cancer.

There is probably not a single one of us who doesn't know someone who has had cancer and who has personally been touched by the pain and suffering of this dreaded disease.

It is not the purpose of this small book to detail the various types of cancer and the death tolls they exact, but let it suffice to say that lung, colon, prostate and breast cancers kill more Americans than any other forms.

While most of us think that cancer is an inherited disease, science shows us that fewer than 2% of all cancer is related to genetics (broken or mutated genes). That means 98% of cancer is caused by something else.

That "something else" has opened a whole new science called epigenetics, meaning literally "above genetics."

The good news is that we have far more control over our epigenetics than genetics.

Renowned scientist Ajay Goel, Ph.D., of the Gastrointestinal

Cancer Research Laboratory at the Baylor Research Institute at Dallas, is at the forefront of epigenetic research.

He explains a complex science in simple terms: "Everything we do from the day we are born, everything we eat, drink and are exposed to in our environment has an indirect but strong influence on our genetics. As we age and grow, it is very natural that some of the genes tend to get turned off as a consequence of our eating habits, exercise regimens and exposure to toxic environmental stresses. Doing the right thing in this regard can help us keep our genes healthy."

So, when we don't eat correctly or exercise and are exposed to toxins, damage to genes takes place and disease occurs.

"Fortunately, unlike genetic defects, epigenetic alterations have a unique characteristic that these changes are reversible," says Dr. Goel.

"In other words, although we can do nothing if we are born with a defective gene, it is certainly within our reach to keep our genomes healthy and we can even reverse some of the epigenetic changes by eating right and with regular consumption of health-promoting natural dietary botanicals and herbals," he explains.

Here's where curcumin comes into the cancer picture.

"Every cell in our bodies has a finite life span," says Dr. Goel. "We have genes in our bodies that govern this natural process of cell death. But sometimes those genes go into a deep slumber, allowing cells to continue to live and reproduce long beyond their time, creating cancerous tumors."

Curcumin has been scientifically proven to actually "wake up" those sleeping genes, telling cancer cells it is time to die and stopping the growth of cancerous tumors.

Dr. Goel and his team have produced ground-breaking research that promises to change the way we think about cancer and how it is treated—and curcumin certainly has a strong role in this change.

It almost goes without saying that the anti-inflammatory and antioxidant powers of curcumin are the foundation of its ability to prevent and treat cancer, since cancer is caused by inflammation and by oxidative stress, meaning, among other things, that DNA has been damaged, impairing the ability of cells to reproduce perfectly.

The staid and highly respected MD Anderson Cancer Center has expressed uncharacteristic enthusiasm about curcumin's anticancer properties in a 2003 statement by researchers published in the journal *Anticancer Research*:

"Extensive research over the last 50 years has indicated it can prevent and treat cancer . . . Curcumin can suppress tumor initiation, promotion and metastasis."

Let's take a look at the large body of research that proves curcumin's effectiveness at preventing and fighting cancer:

Breast cancer cells.

Blocks carcinogenic substances: We're all exposed to carcinogens on a daily basis from auto exhausts, air pollution, food packaging, pesticides and a broad spectrum of substances with which we cannot avoid contact. Curcumin apparently blocks those carcinogens, preventing them from causing the cellular damage that ultimately results in cancer.

Stops invasion: Cancer cells invade normal tissue with the help of certain enzymes called matrix metalloproteinase. Curcumin slows or stops the activity of this enzyme, helping halt the spread of cancerous cells.

Cuts off tumor blood supply: Invasive tumors are fed by their own specially developed network of blood vessels through a process called angiogenesis. Curcumin slows the ability of these tumors to create their blood supply, eventually starving and killing the abnormal clusters of cells.

Convinces cancerous cells to die: As Dr. Goel points out, "sleeping genes" interfere with the cancer cells' natural life and death cycle called apoptosis. Cancer cells quite literally turn off the signal that it is time to die. Curcumin actually turns *on* that signal, telling the cancer cells to die, so the tumors eventually die, too. Dr. Goel is currently engaged in more research on the sleeping gene mechanism.

These are the basic ways that curcumin works to prevent and stop cancer. There are literally dozens of studies that show curcumin's effectiveness against specific types of cancer.

Here's a list of types of cancer for which curcumin has been scientifically validated as a preventive or treatment:

Breast	Head and neck	Oral
Cervical	Leukemia	Ovarian
Colorectal	Lung	Prostate
Gastrointestinal	Lymphoma	Sarcoma
Genitourinary	Melanoma	Squamous cell

As a final word, even the famed Sloan-Kettering Cancer Center is on the curcumin bandwagon, endorsing an anticancer cocktail mixed with another known cancer preventive, green tea.

As yet unpublished animal studies show strong evidence that curcumin, administered in tandem with more traditional anticancer drugs, reduces the toxicity of those drugs and improves their effectiveness. Three human studies are now underway combining curcumin with certain types of chemotherapy drugs commonly used to treat breast and colon cancers. I'm eagerly awaiting more information on this exciting development. However, there have been several promising studies on the ability of curcumin to improve the effectiveness of many types of chemo and radiation therapy by making the cancer cells more sensitive to these treatments. However, please discuss with your integrative health professional how best to use curcumin if you are currently undergoing cancer treatment.

CONCLUSION

While the scientific evidence in favor of curcumin for all of the diseases mentioned in this book is impressive, the quality of proof that curcumin prevents and treats a wide variety of cancer is truly exceptional.

Cancer prevention alone should be a sufficient incentive to include curcumin in your daily supplement regimen.

CHAPTER 4

Curcumin, Chronic Pain and Arthritis

Virtually all of us experience occasional joint and back pain. With luck, it goes away with time, rest and perhaps an occasional ice pack. Sometimes it does not.

Each year, about 30 million of us visit a doctor complaining of joint pain. Another 40 million or so visit a doctor looking for relief from back pain. Add in 1.5 million people with rheumatoid arthritis, 6.1 million with gout, 5 million with fibromyalgia and 1.5 million broken bones suffered every year by people with osteoporosis and you'll see the magnitude of this painful problem.

Long-term musculoskeletal pain affects your entire being. It drains your energy and contributes to chronic stress, a condition that has myriad negative side effects, including obesity, metabolic disorders, heart disease and perhaps even cancer. Chronic pain is often linked with depression. Who wouldn't be depressed in the face of unrelenting pain?

Joint pain and back pain are most often caused by deterioration of the cartilage that cushion joints (including the spaces between the vertebrae, causing back pain), causing bone to rub against bone and resulting in inflammation and pain. This can be caused by an injury, but most often, it is the result of 40, 50, 60 years or more of wear and tear on the joints.

For most of us, our first remedy is to reach for aspirin, ibuprofen or naproxen. That can be a fatal mistake. NSAIDs (nonsteroidal anti-inflammatory drugs) like aspirin, ibuprofen and naproxen plus a handful of prescription drugs like Celebrex, Anaprox, Feldene and Voltaren can cause serious toxicity problems that require hospitalization for as many as 200,000 Americans each year and kill over 20,000 people annually. Yet 60 million of us use them regularly and doctors still happily prescribe them.

Exciting new human research confirms that curcumin is as effective as some of the most popular non-steroidal anti-inflammatory (NSAID) arthritis drugs, including Voltaren and Celebrex, without the potentially life-threatening side effects. A combination formula of BCM-95® Curcumin and a special form of the herb boswellia called BosPure® was found to be more effective in pain relief and provided better mobility and longer walking times without pain for people with knee osteoarthritis, than the prescription drug celecoxib (generic form of Celebrex), the number one prescribed osteoarthritis drug. This study was just published in December of 2011 in the journal *Osteoarthritis and Cartilage*.

NSAIDs relieve inflammation by inhibiting the activity of an inflammation-causing enzyme called COX-2. That's all well and good, but they also inhibit a companion enzyme called COX-1, which protects the lining of the digestive tract and blood vessels. Therefore, without adequate COX-1 protection, you may have ulcers and leaking of the blood vessels.

THE GOLDEN KNIGHT RIDES AGAIN

It shouldn't surprise you that curcumin and its formidable anti-inflammatory powers offer an effective and safe alternative to these dangerous NSAIDs. Curcumin inhibits the COX-2 enzyme but does not affect healthy levels of COX-1.

Inflammation causes pain, so if you relieve inflammation, you relieve pain. Not only does curcumin relieve inflammation and pain, it can actually help rebuild worn cartilage, restoring joints to their youthful flexibility. Curcumin is also such a potent antioxidant that it can actually help repair the oxidative damage caused by inflammation.

Medicine Hunter Chris Kilham, who has conducted medical research in more than 20 countries, is sometimes called "The Indiana Jones of Natural Medicine." He says curcumin deserves "superstar status" among healing plants. "Medicines should heal, not hurt. They should promote life, not take it away. In part, due to disappointment with drugs, and in part due to a belief that natural remedies are safer than most pharmaceuticals, many people seek natural remedies to alleviate pain. But where do they look? Enter curcumin, a derivative of turmeric root, that literally can erase pain quickly and powerfully, without negative effects," says Kilham.

The research is very impressive:

Reduce inflammation: Biological indicators of inflammation were reduced by as much as 99% with curcumin, offering almost complete relief for chronic pain sufferers and providing powerful promise for prevention and treatment of other diseases caused by inflammation.

Cartilage regeneration: Not only does curcumin help reduce the inflammation, it actually helps prevent the breakdown of cartilage (the cushions between joints), preventing arthritis from developing or worsening, as shown by Canadian researchers. At least one study shows that curcumin can help build new cartilage cells, reversing what was once thought to be an incurable degenerative disease.

Pain relief: An Italian study showed that people diagnosed with knee osteoarthritis were able to reduce their need for NSAIDs by 63% when they took curcumin. As a welcome side effect in this study, it was discovered that curcumin produced a 16-fold *reduction* in participants' blood levels of CRP, the protein that indicates high levels of inflammation, which also predicts a high risk for heart attack.

Once again curcumin has proven to be superior to commonly used pharmaceuticals in relieving joint pain and increasing walking time among people with knee osteoarthritis. In a 2011 study published in the journal *Osteoarthritis and Cartilage,* patients who took a 500 mg blend of BCM-95® Curcumin and BosPure®

boswellia twice daily had significantly better pain relief than those who took 100 mg of celecoxib (generic form of Celebrex) twice a day. The curcumin-boswellia blend equaled celecoxib in improved joint flexibility. However, Celebrex has serious negative side effects, including irregular heartbeat, depression, increased risk of heart attack and stroke, stomach and intestinal bleeding, chest pain, ulcers, severe abdominal pain, jaundice, one-sided weakness and more. I cannot for the life of me understand why anyone would take this drug when natural curcumin and boswellia offer better results and no serious side effects at all.

Rheumatoid arthritis: A landmark 2006 study from the University of Arizona takes the idea of inflammation a step further with the finding that curcumin might *prevent* rheumatoid arthritis, an autoimmune disease. Another study showed that curcumin was at least as effective as one commonly prescribed pain reliever for rheumatoid arthritis.

The most recent research published in the journal *Phytotherapy Research* in March 2012 shows that people with rheumatoid arthritis taking 500 mg of BCM-95® Curcumin twice daily had as much pain relief and improved mobility as those who received diclofenac sodium (generic form of the drug Voltaren, a pharmaceutical commonly prescribed for people with rheumatoid arthritis) with a vastly superior safety profile. Side effects associated with Voltaren include ulcers, bleeding in the stomach and gastrointestinal tract, life-threatening blood loss, irregular heartbeat, chest pain, fainting and many others. No side effects were reported in the patients who received BCM-95® Curcumin.

CONCLUSION

If you suffer from occasional or continuous joint pain, like most of us, you'll discover that curcumin offers short- and long-term relief. You can find the same kind of pain relief as my sister, who has suffered from chronic back pain for decades and found relief with her first dose of curcumin.

CHAPTER 5

Curcumin and Diabetes

Type 2 diabetes is the disease of the Western lifestyle. This disease, once known as adult-onset diabetes, was considered the province of the over-50 crowd. You know the ones I mean, the ones with the potbellies, vegging out in front of the TV, munching on Doritos chased with half a gallon of Rocky Road.

Now it is the disease of teens raised on Big Macs and gallons of Coke, 20-somethings with high cholesterol, 30-somethings with erectile dysfunction and 40-somethings with coronary bypasses.

Type 1 diabetes is usually diagnosed in children and is characterized by a malfunctioning pancreas that does not produce sufficient quantities of the body's own insulin to properly utilize the natural sugars in food.

Type 2 diabetes, on the other hand, is a lifestyle disease. Scientifically, it is characterized by the body's inability to respond to the insulin produced by the pancreas. This is called insulin resistance.

The American Diabetes Association reports that 25.8 million Americans suffer from the disease, 7 million of them undiagnosed. Another 79 million are considered "prediabetic," meaning they have some blood sugar malfunction.

It's important to note that the vast majority of people with type 2 diabetes are obese. Alarmingly, the number of people with diabetes in the U.S. has increased by 76% in the last 20 years in pace with the increase in obesity.

Just having to live with blood glucose testing, dietary restrictions and diabetes meds with a wide variety of side effects is only the tip of the diabetes iceberg.

DEADLY COMPLICATIONS

The complications of diabetes are daunting:

- Heart disease is reported as a cause of death in 68% of people with diabetes aged 65 and over.

- People with diabetes have a 2 to 4 times greater chance of dying of heart disease or stroke than those without the disease.

- High blood pressure is reported in 67% of those with diabetes.

- Diabetes is the leading cause of new cases of blindness in people aged 29 to 74.

- Kidney failure attributed to diabetes accounts for 44% of all new cases. In 2008, the latest year for which statistics are available, more than 202,000 people with end-stage kidney disease due to diabetes were living on dialysis or with a kidney transplant.

- Nerve damage is experienced by 60 to 70% of people with diabetes, often causing erectile dysfunction in men.

- Diabetes causes circulatory problems that led to 65,700 lower limb amputations in diabetics in 2008.

- Diabetes is listed as a contributing cause of death in more than 231,000 deaths.

Science now generally accepts that diabetes is an inflammatory condition, as is obesity. As you might well imagine, this is where curcumin comes into the picture.

THE GOLDEN KNIGHT REDUX

Remember the role of free radical oxygen molecules as underlying causes of most disease processes from Chapter 1?

Curcumin's antioxidant and anti-inflammatory properties are especially applicable to diabetes and its complications.

Here's what the studies show curcumin can do:

Reduce glucose production in the liver: A Japanese study shows that curcumin has the ability to reduce the liver's natural production of glucose, which in healthy people is balanced by the pancreas's production of insulin to keep glucose levels steady.

Keep glucose out of red blood cells: Scientists treated red blood cells to mimic diabetes, then exposed them to curcumin for just 24 hours. The results: Curcumin normalized the cells in terms of sugar processing and prevented the formation of the fatty globules that clog arteries.

Prevent the development of diabetes: A Columbia University study showed that mice with a predisposition toward diabetes and obesity given daily doses of curcumin were less likely to develop impaired blood sugar, insulin resistance and full-blown diabetes than those that did not receive curcumin.

Lower blood sugar, increase insulin: Indian researchers found that curcumin contains a particularly powerful antioxidant, tetrahydro-curcumin, which lowers blood sugars, increases insulin in the bloodstream (meaning existing insulin is being properly used) and protects against fatty deposits in the arteries indicative of heart disease that is very common in people with diabetes. Through its anti-inflammatory action, several studies show that curcumin can result in better blood sugar control and, therefore, a small, but significant decrease in body weight and fat, potentially reducing the risk of Type 2 diabetes.

Promote wound healing: Curcumin also helps in the process of wound healing, something that is especially important to people with diabetes since their wound-healing capabilities are often impaired, leading to infection and amputations. Curcumin should be used at the time when the skin is beginning to re-form around the wound and new skin is being laid down.

Protect kidneys: Curcumin has also been found to protect the kidneys, which we know are vulnerable in people with diabetes, and to help prevent glaucoma and cataracts, common complications among people with diabetes.

Reduce liver inflammation: Animal studies show that BCM-95® Curcumin actually reduced liver inflammation, making the livers of the treated obese animals (cats in this case) behave like the livers of non-obese animals. Yes, these are "only" animal studies, but experts like Dr. Ajay Goel of Baylor think that it is logical that BCM-95® will have similar effects on humans, reducing fatty liver and obesity, among the greatest risks for diabetes.

Reverse diabetes: Probably the most exciting study came from Egypt in 2008, when researchers discovered curcumin and a bone marrow transplant reversed diabetes in mice with the disease. Researchers theorized that the anti-inflammatory and antioxidant properties of curcumin enhanced the ability of the bone marrow transplant to regenerate insulin-producing cells.

CONCLUSION

The evidence is abundantly clear: Curcumin has profound effects against one of the most deadly diseases of our time. Its pathways of action are widely varied, and it is effective against a number of the complications of diabetes as well. While doctors are not yet ready to tell every person with diabetes to take curcumin, they are probably behind the research curve. If I had diabetes, wild horses couldn't keep me away from my curcumin. I don't have diabetes, but curcumin is still a staple of my supplement regimen.

CHAPTER 6

Curcumin and Memory: Alzheimer's and Dementia

Brain health is at the core of who we are as humans.

If you have a healthy brain, you have an inquiring mind, you are engaged in the world around you, and you communicate clearly with others and form nurturing relationships.

Brain chemistry malfunctions take place when, for unknown reasons, brain cells begin to die, resulting in impaired memory, also known as dementia. It is a disease in itself and is not a normal consequence of aging.

Alzheimer's disease is probably the best-known form of dementia, accounting for 50 to 70% of all cases of dementia, so the terms Alzheimer's and dementia are often used interchangeably. Many people with Alzheimer's show signs of dementia caused by strokes or mini-strokes called transient ischemic accidents (TIAs) as well.

Dementia can also be caused by chemical exposures, other neurological diseases like Parkinson's and Creutzfeldt-Jakob (mad cow disease), long-term depression, multiple strokes, AIDS, chronic drug use, infections and toxic side effects of medications. It can also be caused by head injuries, as we've learned through recent media coverage of compromised brain function in professional football players and boxers who are exposed to relentless blows to the head. For the most part these, like Alzheimer's, are incurable and irreversible. Conventional medicine has little to offer in terms of treatment.

There are also forms of dementia that can be treated and potentially reversed, including those caused by a blood clot on the brain, a tumor that can be removed, hypothyroidism, hypoglycemia and vitamin B12 deficiency.

It is very difficult to diagnose dementia or to differentiate the specific disease called Alzheimer's, so if you or someone close to you is showing signs of memory loss, it is essential to make a thorough investigation to determine if the dementia is caused by one of the factors that can be treated and reversed.

THE LONG GOODBYE

Over time, Alzheimer's inevitably affects memory, thinking and behavior. People with Alzheimer's frequently experience personality changes, anxiety, anger and may even become combative and violent.

Alzheimer's has often been called "The Long Goodbye," because it takes such a terrible physical and emotional toll on its victims and their families, usually for years on end.

Curcumin stimulates electrical communication between brain cells.

The downhill memory slide takes its victims from normal competency with occasional memory lapses to the loss of the ability to function in the normal world to inevitable death with no apparent mindfulness. Sadly, conventional medicine offers no really effective treatment. The few pharmaceuticals on the market have minimal effects even in slowing the progression of the disease.

The National Institutes of Health estimates that more than 5 million Americans have Alzheimer's. Most of them are over 60, although there is an increasing rate of early onset Alzheimer's that can begin as early as the 30s. The frightening statistic is that if you're lucky to live to the age of 85, you have a 50-50 chance of developing dementia.

Alzheimer's is inevitably a fatal disease, but it rarely kills quickly. Mercifully, people with dementia often have other diseases that take them away before the terrible onset of late-stage dementia.

BIOLOGY OF ALZHEIMER'S

Here's a little painless biology that explains how normal brain cells work:

I like to think of neurons, dendrites and synapses as an electrical system in the brain through which thought processes and conscious and unconscious biological functions take place. Neurons, the brain cells, grow large finger-like projections called dendrites that function very much like wiring in an electrical system. Each neuron has at least one dendrite in and another out in this electrical grid that sends a charge to the next dendrite across a tiny space called a synapse. Scientists once thought that we are born with all of the neurons and dendrites we will ever possess, but they've recently learned that over our lifetimes we can grow new neurons and even expand our network of dendrites exponentially in a process called neurogenesis. Some neurons may have hundreds or even thousands of dendrites.

Continuing our analogy of the electrical wiring system, you can see that if one wire becomes damaged, thousands of alternative "electrical" pathways can allow the system to continue to function without impairment.

How do you grow more dendrites and refresh your neuron supply? No one is really sure, but there is evidence that the more you challenge your brain, the more extensive your neuronal network will be.

Another process characteristic of Alzheimer's is the formation of beta-amyloid plaques and tangles. The beta-amyloid plaques are made of protein that accumulates around the neurons rather than being eliminated by the body, as they are in a healthy person, thereby damaging the function of the brain.

In addition, tangled proteins called tau fibers inside the neuron further impair the mental process.

These plaques and tangles and disrupted neuronal function most often occur in the hippocampus, the lower part of the human brain that is responsible for memory. For unknown reasons, Alzheimer's and other forms of dementia frequently affect the area of the hippocampus that controls short-term memory. That's why Grandma may have no idea what she ate for breakfast, but she can recount in great detail the guest list and menu from a dinner party 30 years ago.

Alzheimer's is usually staged in seven levels, the seventh stage being inevitably fatal when the neuronal network has failed to the extent that bodily functions that require little or no thought (like swallowing or coughing) become so impaired that their failure is life threatening.

The average life expectancy for someone with Alzheimer's is 8 to 10 years from the onset of symptoms, although it may take several years to obtain a diagnosis.

YES, IT CAN BE INHERITED—OR NOT

There is a genetic component of Alzheimer's, both with late onset and the increasingly diagnosed early onset. Scientists have identified the genetic component, called APOE that can forecast a person's risk for the disease later in life. But the presence of the APOE gene is not at all predictive that the carrier of the gene will develop the disease. In fact, many people who do have the APOE gene never develop Alzheimer's, and conversely, many without the genetic component do develop it.

Baby Boomers experiencing the emotionally and financially draining farewell of their grandparents and parents are understandably concerned about their own futures.

Prevention and slowing mental deterioration in the early stages of Alzheimer's is where BCM-95® Curcumin may be the most helpful, according to pioneering Alzheimer's researcher Ralph Martins, head of Australia's Sir James McCusker Unit for Alzheimer's Disease Research for more than 20 years.

For most people, Dr. Martins says, "I think curcumin should play an important role in slowing down the disease or possibly preventing it." He adds, "In terms of curcumin's ability to slow down the progression of preclinical Alzheimer's disease, there is now very strong evidence from animal trials that curcumin markedly lowers the level of beta-amyloid in the brain and does it primarily by affecting its aggregation (clumping of the plaque) and facilitating its clearance (elimination from the body). In addition, curcumin is a powerful antioxidant and thus plays a significant role in reducing brain damage caused by oxidative stress."

Dr. Martins is currently engaged in human studies using BCM-95® Curcumin to verify this preliminary work.

OTHER MEANS OF PREVENTION

Increased physical and mental activities have been shown to keep brain cells active, improve circulation and stave off dementia. Stress management and what the Alzheimer's Research and Prevention Foundation calls "brain aerobics" (challenging your brain to activities outside your norm—think Sudoku or writing haiku) are also important elements in preventing dementia.

Several studies also show the healthy Omega-3 fats from fish are key components in brain health and memory preservation as is a healthy diet rich in antioxidants like berries, green leafy vegetables, nuts, seeds and citrus fruits.

While there are several anti-dementia pharmaceuticals on the market, they do not reverse dementia and they have limited effectiveness in slowing its progress.

THE GOLDEN KNIGHT RIDES AGAIN

Curcumin's unique ability to cross the blood-brain barrier means that it can affect brain chemistry and the survival mechanisms of brain cells (neurons), producing preventive and healing effects that few other nutrients can offer.

Curcumin, and particularly BCM-95® Curcumin, holds great promise for those with dementia and particularly for people with a history of Alzheimer's in their families. There has been extensive research in this area (a search of curcumin+dementia in the National Institutes of Health database turns up 134 studies). The enthusiasm for the results is becoming intense.

Compared to the Western world, there is a much lower rate of Alzheimer's disease in India, where curcumin is eaten in large quantities in the curries that are a staple of the Indian diet. In fact, the rate of Alzheimer's in India among people ages 70 to 79 is about one-quarter of the rate in the U.S. where curcumin is rarely included in the diet.

Even eating a small amount of curcumin seems to have an effect. One study showed better memory among 60- to 93-year-olds who ate curry just once a month than among those who never ate it.

Here's a fascinating story about Indian people who tend to eat curry two or three times a day, so their dietary intake of curcumin is exceptionally high:

Researchers conducting autopsies on the brains of Indians who died of all causes found that there was an unusual yellowish color in their brain stem (hippocampus) tissue. This color, not seen in people of other ethnicities, was taken as proof that curcumin indeed crosses the blood-brain barrier and that large quantities of it are actually absorbed into the brain tissue.

Here are a few of the most interesting research results on curcumin and the brain:

Grow new brain cells: Until recently, scientists believed that it was impossible to grow new brain cells, but they busted that myth with the discovery of neurogenesis, the scientifically validated creation of new brain cells. University of Florida researchers have now confirmed that curcumin stimulates the birth of new neurons, particularly in the hippocampus, the seat of memory in the human brain.

Protect brain cells: Authors of a study published in the journal *Current Alzheimer's Research* were enthusiastic about antioxidant properties of curcumin to prevent brain cell deterioration and death. Inflammatory cells called cytokines have a role in speeding up Alzheimer's, and the abilities of curcumin to inhibit the COX-2 enzyme can help protect those brain cells.

Destroy plaques and tangles: Scientists at UCLA called curcumin "anti-amyloid" for its ability to overcome the beta-amyloid protein that forms the plaques and tangles. They also noted that people with Alzheimer's show signs of inflammation in their brains and credit curcumin's anti-inflammatory properties with an ability to address that problem. Another UCLA animal study showed curcumin supplements reduced substances believed to cause plaque by 43 to 45%. Some researchers have suggested curcumin binds directly to plaques and eliminates them.

The most exciting new research on curcumin, and particularly the BCM-95® formulation, suggests that curcumin helps dissolve those beta-amyloid plaques that are widely believed in the scientific community to cause the neuronal "short-circuit" that results in memory loss indicative of Alzheimer's disease and other forms of dementia.

The 34 participants in this study published in the *Journal of Psychopharmacology* had all been diagnosed with probable or possible Alzheimer's disease based on criteria set by the National

Institute of Neurological and Communicative Disorders and Stroke–Alzheimer Disease and Related Disorders Association. They were given either a placebo or one or four grams of BCM-95® Curcumin. There were few side effects and, interestingly, the most side effects occurred in the placebo group.

Researchers commented on the resulting increased levels of beta-amyloid in the bloodstream as indicative that the beta-amyloid plaque formations in their brains were dissolving and the bloodstream was carrying them away for waste disposal.

In addition, BCM-95® has been selected for study in a groundbreaking, exciting, year-long Australian clinical study searching for ways to prevent or delay the expected declines of Alzheimer's disease, being conducted by renowned Australian researcher Ralph Martins, Ph.D., who directed the study on beta-amyloid plaque mentioned previously on page 30.

As head of the Sir James McCusker Unit for Alzheimer's Disease Research for over 20 years, Director of the Centre of Excellence for Alzheimer's Disease Research and Care, Director and Inaugural Chair for Ageing and Alzheimer's Disease at Edith Cowan University in Perth, Australia, Dr. Martins is working to develop an early diagnostic blood test in order to effectively prevent and/or treat this devastating degenerative brain disease.

In addition, Dr. Martins and his team are working to substantiate their theory that the presence of curcumin in the retina of the eye, when it is bound to the beta-amyloid plaque, may help doctors diagnose Alzheimer's in its earliest stages and perhaps reverse the disease process with more curcumin. I am very excited about Dr. Martins' work and look forward to results that will change the face of Alzheimer's disease, prevention, diagnosis and treatment in the not-too-distant future.

Curcumin studies in animal models of Alzheimer's disease have demonstrated that it can play a significant role in the destruction of beta-amyloid plaque. It is also a powerful antioxidant, with an ORAC value of 1.5 million per 100 grams, as determined by the United States Department of Agriculture (USDA). Other studies have shown that curcumin plays a role in neuronal regeneration. All these properties contribute to its potential utility in addressing this brain disease.

"I chose BCM-95® Curcumin for my human studies because it has published human bioavailability data," says Dr. Martins. "Therefore, I can use a reasonable amount and expect that the serum levels will achieve a therapeutic range for a significant period of time."

Improve memory in people with Alzheimer's: This exciting Indian study explores multiple ways in which curcumin not only prevents Alzheimer's and slows the progression of the disease, but actually improves memory in people already diagnosed with the disease.

Chelating heavy metals: The same Indian study says that curcumin helps eliminate heavy metals from brain cells and shields the cells from heavy metal contamination. These heavy metals have long been implicated in Alzheimer's and dementia.

CONCLUSION

I'm reluctant to use superlatives in a book like this, but I am greatly excited about the power of curcumin to protect the brain and to prevent, treat and even reverse dementia and Alzheimer's through a broad network of chemical pathways. Although I would caution you that most of these studies are done at the cellular level or on animals, and human studies are just getting underway, there are ample reasons for encouragement.

Although doctors are highly unlikely to recommend curcumin for the treatment of these brain-related diseases, if I had a loved one suffering from one of them, I'd be very eager to give highly absorbable BCM-95® Curcumin a try.

CHAPTER 7

Curcumin, Depression and Other Brain Disorders

Curcumin's value in treating dementia and Alzheimer's disease opens the door to its considerable value in treating and preventing a variety of other malfunctions of the brain and the neurotransmitter system.

DEPRESSION

Over a lifetime, 16.5% of the U.S. adult population (18.8 million people) suffers from a major depressive disorder and 30% of those cases are so severe that they impair the ability to work or even to function in the world in normal terms.

We know that women are 70% more likely to develop depression, that Caucasians have a 40% higher risk for depression than African-Americans and that people between the ages of 18 and 29 are at much greater risk of major depressive disorders than people over 60.

Depression affects children as well. Government statistics show 4.7% of 13- to 18-year-olds suffer from severe mood disorders and girls are nearly twice as vulnerable as boys. The rate of teen depression is increasing by an alarming 23% per year.

We're not talking about the occasional day or even days of feeling blue. We're not talking about the normal ups and downs of life, the loss of a relationship, the loss of a job or even the loss of a loved one.

Depressive disorder is a crushing inability to cope with life and the world. Yet only about half of its sufferers get treatment and 80% of the treatment that conventional medicine offers is completely ineffective.

Standard medical treatment for depression is usually a series of antidepressant pharmaceuticals with a high risk of serious side effects and little or no effect. Research shows that antidepressants work for only 35 to 45% of the population, and some figures suggest the effectiveness rate is as low as 30%. Worse yet, antidepressants like Prozac, Paxil and Zoloft have been linked to suicide, violence, psychosis, abnormal bleeding and brain tumors.

What causes depression? Certainly short-term depression can be the result of life events. Long-term trauma, such as sexual abuse and a family history of depression can also be factors.

Dr. Hyla Cass, a cutting-edge integrative physician with a specialty in psychiatry, believes that the cause of depression is often biochemical, an imbalance in brain chemistry.

The answer, says Dr. Cass in her book *Natural Highs: Feel Good All the Time,* is in "a variety of nutrients that both make up and fuel the brain, nervous system and neurotransmitters. So a low mood may have less to do with past trauma or a faulty belief system than with deficient nutrients."

"Mood-lifting serotonin, motivating noradrenaline and sleep-enhancing tryptophan are the neurotransmitters most often deficient in people with depression," says Dr. Cass.

You guessed it: Here comes the Golden Knight on his charger again, offering solutions to brain imbalances that are at the foundation of major depression. Not only does curcumin enhance noradrenaline and tryptophan levels, but it also increases the production of dopamine, another neurotransmitter that controls emotional response and the ability to experience pleasure and pain.

Numerous studies underscore curcumin's ability to improve levels of neurotransmitters and thereby improve mood.

Many people stumble on curcumin's antidepressant action when they take it for another condition, most typically to address joint pain. The action is so subtle that some users have written that they didn't realize their depression had disappeared until they stopped taking curcumin and the depression returned.

Here are highlights of the research on curcumin and depression:

Increases serotonin and dopamine levels: Several studies support curcumin's ability to boost mood by increasing levels of mood-enhancing neurotransmitters. At least one study adds that curcumin combined with some antidepressant prescription drugs improves their effectiveness.

Acts like pharmaceutical drugs without the risks: Exciting new research shows that BCM-95® Curcumin is as effective as the popular antidepressant pharmaceuticals Prozac (fluoxetine) and Tofranil (imipramine), without the side effects associated with the pharmaceutical drugs that include weight gain and loss, increased depression and increased suicidal tendencies. Another interesting finding published in 2011 showed that BCM-95® Curcumin did nothing to increase the effectiveness of the two pharmaceutical antidepressants, but did just as well as each of them on its own. The bottom line: If you suffer from depression, it is worth a try to go with BCM-95® Curcumin, with the permission of your health care professional. Please don't stop taking your antidepressants cold turkey because it can cause some serious side effects like dramatic moods swings, a worsening of the underlying depression or other condition, extremely vivid dreams, aggression and suicidal tendencies.

Generates new brain cells: Curcumin can actually help in the formation of new nerve cells, called neurogenesis, helping create a healthy balance of the numerous neurotransmitters needed for a healthy brain, better memory and a positive mood.

Antioxidant and anti-inflammatory mood improvement: Indian researchers are clearly enthusiastic about curcumin. Several studies further the body of evidence in favor of curcumin's positive effects on mood.

OTHER BRAIN-PROTECTIVE FUNCTIONS OF CURCUMIN

Curcumin's ability to relieve depression and dementia are considerable, but there's more in the realm of scientific research on curcumin's brain-protective effects:

Blocks brain tumor formation: Researchers in New York discovered that injected curcumin blocks the formation of cancerous brain tumors in mice.

Anti-convulsant: An animal study from India found that curcumin supplements stop epileptic seizures.

Protects brain cells from stroke damage: Oxygen deprivation is the main cause of post-stroke brain damage and disability. A University of Missouri animal study showed that injected curcumin given for two months after a stroke greatly diminished the death of brain cells. Another study showed that after a stroke, curcumin helped prevent damage to the all-important blood-brain barrier, minimizing the risk of infection and other types of brain damage.

Counters effects of traumatic brain injury: UCLA animal researchers found that a diet high in curcumin greatly reduced brain damage and cognitive impairment after a traumatic brain injury.

Treatment for Parkinson's disease: Parkinson's disease is a degenerative disease of the central nervous system that includes movement-related impairment, including shaking, slowness of movement and rigidity of limbs. In its advanced state, Parkinson's can include dementia and behavioral problems.

Modern medicine treats the symptoms of Parkinson's, since there is no known cure.

Inflammation is certainly a part of Parkinson's, and we already know that curcumin is a powerful anti-inflammatory and antioxidant. In addition, 2012 research from the Northeast Ohio Medical University suggests that curcumin has neuroprotective elements as well, particularly in containing the protein accumulations like the plaques and tangles found in Alzheimer's. Researchers in that study said, "Curcumin possesses therapeutic potential in the amelioration of a host of neurodegenerative ailments as evidenced by its antioxidant, anti-inflammatory and anti-protein aggregation effects."

Who knows what the future holds, but this research may eventually show curcumin's value in treating other neurodegenerative diseases like multiple sclerosis and ALS.

In another study, Indian researchers concluded that curcumin holds therapeutic potential for people with Parkinson's disease because of its antioxidant properties, especially those that help rebuild glutathione levels in cells, enhancing nutrient metabolism and immune response.

CONCLUSION

If you or a loved one suffer from depression, or other brain disorders mentioned in this chapter, run—don't walk—to your nearest health food store and get yourself some BCM-95® Curcumin. You have nothing to risk and everything to gain.

Next step: If you are taking prescription antidepressants, schedule an appointment with your doctor. Show him or her this book and ask how to wean yourself from the drugs so you can determine if side-effect free curcumin will work better for you.

CHAPTER 8

Curcumin and Digestive Disorders

Time after time, curcumin has proven its value in treating a wide variety of digestive disorders, largely because of its anti-inflammatory effects.

Digestive disorders range from mild indigestion to life-controlling irritable bowel syndrome to life-threatening diseases like ulcerative colitis and colorectal cancer.

Each year, 62 million Americans are diagnosed with some form of digestive disorder.

Irritable bowel syndrome, a complex and unpredictable basket of painful problems ranging from diarrhea to constipation and cramping, bloating and pain, goes largely undiagnosed with an estimated 75% of sufferers not getting medical treatment at all.

Colorectal cancer kills about 150,000 people every year, and ulcerative colitis and Crohn's disease make life a living hell for 140,000 Americans.

Liver disease is included in this category because of the liver's key role in the digestive process.

HERE COMES THE GOLDEN KNIGHT AGAIN

Because inflammation is a major factor in all digestive disorders, curcumin is predictably very effective in helping prevent, treat and heal many digestive problems.

Herbalists consider curcumin to be a digestive and a bitter, which means it helps ease digestion and aids liver function.

It also stimulates bile production in the liver and gallbladder and improves the ability to digest fats.

Here's a listing of various digestive disorders and how curcumin can help:

Ulcerative colitis: A Japanese study, which involved human subjects, a rarity in curcumin research to this point, suggests curcumin supplements are a safe way of preventing recurrences of the disease and reducing the side effects, which include severe bleeding, ruptured colon, dehydration and liver disease in the small intestine.

Crohn's disease: Researchers at the MD Anderson Cancer Center in Houston recommend we "get back to our roots" and take advantage of the anti-inflammatory effects of curcumin for many dis-

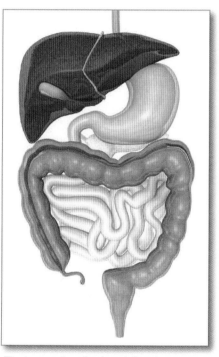

The human liver (top) and digestive system.

eases, including Crohn's, an inflammatory disease usually affecting the large and small intestines. Crohn's and ulcerative colitis are sometimes called inflammatory bowel disease.

Colon cancer: We've already examined curcumin's anticancer properties in Chapter 3, but it's worth mentioning it again here. A landmark study from the American Health Foundation shows that curcumin interferes with the process by which malignant colon tumors develop, stopping them before they become dangerous.

Irritable bowel syndrome: Irritable bowel syndrome is an unpleasant cluster of problems that fluctuate between diarrhea and constipation with abdominal cramps, bloating and gas in the mix. A study from the Medical College of Wisconsin helps us understand better the anti-inflammatory capabilities of curcumin, which stop the growth of additional blood vessels to feed the inflamed area in the digestive tract. This process, called angiogenesis, is also part of the process by which cancerous tumors get their blood supply, enabling them to grow.

Familial adenomatous polyposis: In a study, published in the *Journal of Clinical Gastroenterology and Hepatology,* five patients with an inherited form of precancerous polyps in the lower bowel known as familial adenomatous polyposis (FAP) were treated with regular doses of curcumin and quercetin (another powerful antioxidant found in onions and garlic) during an average of six months. The average number of polyps dropped 60.4 percent, and the average size dropped by 50.9 percent.

Liver damage: An interesting Finnish animal study involved feeding rats a diet that simulated high alcohol consumption. Animals given curcumin at the same time had none of the signs of liver damage normally associated with alcoholism. Researchers theorize that curcumin blocks a molecule called NFkB, which is responsible for inflammation and tissue death. Another study showed that animals with 70% of their livers removed regenerated new liver tissue in as little as 24 hours with the help of curcumin.

CONCLUSION

Once again, curcumin proves its considerable value in fighting inflammation with remarkable results in treating, preventing and stopping the progress of a variety of digestive disorders. The results in treating and preventing liver disease, a potentially fatal affliction, are even more remarkable.

CHAPTER 9

Curcumin and Other Diseases

Looking back at the previous chapters, it seems like there is nothing that curcumin can't prevent or treat. While that's not exactly true, there are several other diseases for which curcumin is highly effective, yet they don't fall neatly into the categories of the other chapters. Nevertheless, they are well worth mentioning.

So here's the "grab bag" of other ways curcumin can be enormously helpful in protecting:

Lungs: Existing drugs have not been shown to be effective in the treatment of lung conditions resulting from occupational and environmental exposures to mineral dusts, airborne pollutants, cigarette smoke, chemotherapy, radiotherapy and other causes of acute and chronic inflammatory lung disease. Several animal studies show that curcumin minimizes lung injury and fibrosis caused by radiation, chemotherapeutic drugs and toxic substances. The researchers also note that studies support the conclusion that curcumin plays a protective role in chronic obstructive pulmonary disease, acute lung injury, acute respiratory distress syndrome and allergic asthma. A recent animal study from the United Arab Emirates confirms the usefulness of curcumin in protecting against the toxic effects of air pollution.

Kidneys: When Indian researchers artificially induced kidney disease in animals, they found that curcumin protected them from

Immune system: white blood cells attack viral invaders.

the toxic buildup that occurs when kidneys can no longer filter the blood. The study also showed that the antioxidants in curcumin protected kidneys against injury.

Eyes: Another Indian study showed that the growth of cataracts in animals with diabetes was significantly slowed when the animals were given curcumin supplements. Researchers theorize that this same protection can be extended to human cataracts that occur when the lens of the eye becomes cloudy. It is common in older people.

Want more? Here is a handful of other diseases that curcumin may help treat or prevent:

Obesity: Obesity is such a huge problem that it probably deserves its own chapter or even its own book. Two-thirds of Americans are overweight, of which one-third are obese. Anything that can help with weight control is welcome. Through its anti-inflammatory action, several studies show that curcumin can result in better blood sugar control and, therefore, a small but significant decrease in body weight and fat. Perhaps more important, it also increases levels of a protein called adiponectin that are usually low in obese people. By raising adiponectin levels, normal weight can return. Curcumin also helps cut off blood supply to excess fat cells, reducing their size and number.

Recent research published in the *British Journal of Nutrition* in late 2011 showed that BCM-95® Curcumin reduced liver inflammation, neutralizing the risk for a fatty liver associated with obesity. So, not only does curcumin help keep weight and blood sugar under control, it can reduce the inflammatory marker for potentially fatal liver disease and lessens the risk for a wide variety of diseases, including diabetes, heart disease and cancer.

Multiple sclerosis: This progressive neurological disease eventually leads to complete disability. Researchers theorize that the same properties in curcumin that protect brain cells may also be helpful in protecting the muscle fibers that are affected by multiple sclerosis (MS). In a Vanderbilt animal study, animals with an MS-like illness showed no signs of the disease after being treated with curcumin while those that did not get curcumin became paralyzed.

Immune system: In particular, studies on HIV show that curcumin slows the ability of the virus to duplicate itself and spread, reducing the viral load on people whose immune systems are already severely compromised. This human study reduced the viral load in 57.8% of the participants. In addition, a Kenyan epidemiological study of people of Indian descent (who eat curry) and those of African descent (who don't eat curry) showed that those of African descent were far more likely to contract HIV.

CONCLUSION

This chapter demonstrates the scope of the potential for curcumin to create profound biological changes and enormous benefits to human health. As mentioned in earlier chapters, there are few human studies. Most of the studies are lab studies on cells or animals, and it is not certain that they can translate to human benefits. Yet the promise is so great that it is well worth adding curcumin, the right kind of curcumin, to your daily supplement regimen. In the next chapter, I'll let you know how and why to get the right kind of curcumin.

CHAPTER 10

BCM-95®: The Super Absorbable, Scientifically Validated Curcumin

The promise of curcumin and its vast effects on health are beyond exciting.

It's also important to remember that turmeric is the parent plant, but curcumin is extracted from the rhizomes of turmeric. Curcumin is a potent healing medicine.

Yet there is one factor that puts a damper on the excitement: Ordinary curcumin is poorly absorbed by the human body. In scientific terms, this means it has limited bioavailability.

But that is *ordinary* curcumin. One company, EuroPharma Inc., has found an *extraordinary* form of highly absorbable curcumin. The curcumin extract, BCM-95®, was developed by a team of respected research scientists. BCM-95® Curcumin is an ingredient in many products sold in health food stores by EuroPharma under the brand name *Terry Naturally* (named after EuroPharma founder Terry Lemerond). It is also found in the EuroMedica brand, sold only in the offices of health care professionals.

A recently completed analysis of curcumin products with enhanced absorption shows that blood levels of BCM-95®, a natural 100% curcumin product, are as much as 10 times higher than other forms of curcumin and stay in the bloodstream for 8 to 12 hours, far longer than any other form of curcumin tested.

Since the publication of the first edition of this book, two more studies have been published confirming the bio-availability of BCM-95®. The Indian research showed that the BCM-95® Curcumin product was retained in the bloodstream for 12 hours, *at a concentration seven times the blood levels researchers were able to measure for plain curcumin*. This is especially important if you are in pain from an injury or a chronic condition because the blood levels of BCM-95® leaped to ten times that of the plain curcumin in the first two hours after study subjects took it.

"BCM-95® amplifies and potentiates curcumin's effectiveness," explains Ajay Goel, Ph.D., of the Gastrointestinal Cancer Research Lab at Baylor University.

BCM-95® is extracted from turmeric roots grown and hand-harvested in the pesticide- and chemical-free fields of Assam, India. Farmers are paid a fair-trade price for their crops, and profits are being used to build a hospital and a school in the village.

Extracting the curcumin from the turmeric rhizomes is a complex process. The BCM-95® plant in Kochi, India, is a state-of-the-art extraction, drying and pulverizing facility that produces high-quality curcumin standardized to 95% curcuminoids. It is then converted into BCM-95®, a proprietary blend of curcuminoids and essential oil of turmeric. EuroPharma's BCM-95® uses no dangerous solvents, unlike products sold by other companies that contain harsh, dangerous and potentially neurotoxic solvents.

Several studies have proven the enhanced effectiveness of BCM-95®, including:

Depression: There are two studies, one animal study showing BCM-95® is at least as effective as Prozac and Tofranil that has already been published and another human study underway that compares BCM-95® Curcumin to the pharmaceutical antidepressant fluoxetine (generic of Prozac). This is particularly important since pharmaceutical antidepressants in general are notoriously ineffective, only providing relief to about 30 to 40% of people with depression. I expect that when this study is published, the results will be amazing!

Osteoarthritis: The latest published research shows that BCM-95® and BosPure® boswellia were superior to celecoxib, a generic of the osteoarthritis drug Celebrex for relief of joint pain.

Rheumatoid arthritis: A study comparing BCM-95® and diclofenac sodium, a pharmaceutical used for rheumatoid arthritis pain and sold under the brand names Cataflam and Voltaren has been published, and it was shown that the group taking 500 mg of BCM-95® curcumin twice daily reported less pain than the diclofenac sodium (Voltaren) group. Nobody withdrew from the curcumin group, but over 14% withdrew from the drug group due to adverse effects.

Alzheimer's disease: Possibly the most exciting study on curcumin's effects on human subjects with mild cognitive impairment is currently underway in Australia. In this study, 160 people with this disorder are being followed for a year to determine to what degree BCM-95® Curcumin slows the progression of the disease. A study from a few years ago on BCM-95® and people with Alzheimer's disease showed that this special curcumin potentially increased the destruction of beta-amyloid plaque, a contributing feature to Alzheimer's damaging brain effects. The results were measured by examining markers found in the bloodstream that indicated beta-amyloid destruction. Human studies on BCM-95® Curcumin are now under way and the results are likely to be paradigm shifting for the prevention and treatment of Alzheimer's.

There are also three ongoing studies of BCM-95® and BosPure® boswellia, another anti-inflammatory herb, exploring antioxidant and liver-protective properties; a study on curcumin in combination with anti-seizure drugs in reduced seizure activity and memory retention; and a human trial on its ability to prevent cancer in premalignant lesions in the mouth.

Several other studies are in the planning stages, one looking at BCM-95®'s role in treating knee osteoarthritis and another study on its ability to preserve cognitive function.

BCM-95® FORMULAS: RECOMMENDED BY DR. MCBARRON

BCM-95® is available in three formulations, each with a specific effect.

Curamin®

Curamin is a blend of curcumin BCM-95®, inflammation-relieving boswellia (BosPure®), DLPA (a form of the amino acid phenylalanine, which increases levels of endorphins, the "feel good" neurotransmitters) and nattokinase (an enzyme that helps improve micro-circulation).

This blend provides a safer and more effective pain-relieving effect than most prescription drugs and OTC medications. In fact, the BCM-95® Curcumin in this formula was proven clinically to be more effective than the pharmaceutical drug celecoxib, the generic form of Celebrex, a joint pain medication with many potentially serious side effects.

Many people using Curamin for the first time will get excellent pain relief within 20 to 45 minutes. Because of different levels of pain and location, some people may have to wait several days for pain relief. Curamin does not have any serious known contraindications with medication, but, of course, check with your doctor or pharmacist if you need more specific information. Curamin can be used along with other pain-relieving medications. It does not cause stomach, liver or kidney damage and can be used long term.

The recommended dosage is three capsules daily, but the dosage can be adjusted based on the needs of the individual. Usually 90% of individuals will experience superior results within seven days. If you do not have excellent relief, take six capsules a day for a week and then reduce the dosage until you find the amount that keeps you comfortable.

A small percentage of people who do not respond to Curamin alone will find an excellent response when they take three capsules a day of Curamin along with one or two capsules a day of Arthocin, EuroPharma's joint pain formula. Arthocin includes some additional joint-rebuilding ingredients, like a unique devil's claw herb that has been shown to increase production of hyaluronic acid by chondrocytes (soft tissue cells in the joint) by 41%. This is a *powerful* combination to help lubricate joints. There are no known serious prescription or over-the-counter interactions with Curamin and/or Arthocin.

Curamin® PM—Sleep Away Your Pain!

Curamin PM is an excellent pain reliever and natural sleep aid. For those who cannot sleep due to pain, Curamin PM will help as a natural, gentle aid for sleep with the dual action of pain reduction. Since the body's repair and rebuild functions take place in deep sleep, individuals who have disrupted sleep do not heal as quickly. Curamin PM contains many of the same pain ingredients as Curamin, but with the added benefits of P-5-P to increase serotonin levels and melatonin to aid in regulating sleep cycles.

Dosage: Take one or two capsules 30 minutes before bedtime. Some people find excellent results taking two regular Curamin in the morning and two Curamin PM at bedtime. There are no known serious interactions with prescription or over-the-counter medications.

CuraMed®

This highly effective, standardized and concentrated curcumin for inflammation can be used for any inflammatory state: all types of arthritis, Crohn's disease, colitis, bronchitis, asthma, sinusitis, bursitis and tendonitis as well as protecting cellular health. The BCM-95® in CuraMed is a very powerful antioxidant with an ORAC (Oxygen Radical Absorbent Capacity) value of over 1.5 million per 100 grams, as reported by independent third party testing. Compare that antioxidant ranking with blueberries, which are considered to have an ORAC ranking of 6,000 per 100 grams. Not surprisingly, BCM-95® Curcumin is a strong immune enhancer, liver protector and detoxifier.

CuraMed is produced with a unique and patented process that delivers a curcumin that is up to 1,000% more bioavailable than curcumin standardized to 95%. You'd have to take up to *10 capsules* of plain curcumin or up to *500 capsules* of plain turmeric to equal just *one* CuraMed capsule's impact on serum curcumin levels.

The patented process for BCM-95® Curcumin ensures 8 to 12 hours retention in the body at significant levels.

Two capsules daily would equal the quantity used in many clinical studies. The combination of its high antioxidant activity and anti-inflammatory action creates the most powerful solution to support the entire metabolic functioning of the body.

CuraMed comes in two dosages: a 750 mg softgel (standardized to 500 mg of pure curcuminoids) and a 375 mg softgel (standardized to 250 mg of pure curcuminoids). The lower dose is ideal for children and smaller pets, and recommended for maintenance

dosages for adults. Either formulation is extremely effective at a dosage of one to two softgels daily. No serious side effects have been reported at this dosage. As with all other BCM-95® supplements, there are no known serious side effects or interactions with prescription medications.

CuraMed® Brain

Combining the proven effects of BCM-95® Curcumin, vitamin D3, and rosemary and Spanish sage oils, this powerhouse supplement supports healthy memory and focus, shields the brain from free radical damage, and enhances cognitive function.

The highly bioabsorbable BCM-95® Curcumin has been clinically tested to be ten times more absorbable and retained at a meaningful level for a longer time than other curcumin extracts. Curcumin is exceptionally effective in stopping and even reversing inflammation and protecting cells from the oxidative stress that is the source of many diseases associated with aging, including Alzheimer's, dementia, diabetes, heart disease and cancer.

In addition, clinical studies show that vitamin D3 in the levels found in CuraMed® Brain (2,000 IU) is associated with healthy brain function and improved resistance to many brain diseases. Vitamin D partnered with curcumin has been shown in preliminary research to be particularly potent with regards to Alzheimer's disease. Clinical trials show that Spanish sage and rosemary oils improve brain levels of acetylcholine, an important neurotransmitter that diminishes with age and in certain diseases, which in turn can improve memory and recall, improve focus and help protect the brain from damaging free radicals.

However, with these and all supplements, always check with your health care professional before combining them with prescription drugs.

All EuroPharma curcumin formulas are available at quality health food stores and medical professional offices.

CONCLUSION

There are many curcumin and turmeric products on the market, but they are essentially worthless if your body cannot use them.

As you've seen in this book, the healing powers of curcumin are more than impressive. They are stunning. In fact, it is possible they could replace multivitamins as the #1 supplement in your medicine cabinet.

It only makes sense to use a product that is proven to be effective.

References

Chapter 2

Soni KB, Kuttan R. Effect of oral curcumin administration on serum peroxides and cholesterol levels in human volunteers. *Indian J Physiol Pharmacol.* 1992 Oct;36(4):273–275.

Ramaswami G, Chair H et al. Curcumin blocks homocysteine-induced endothelial dysfunction in porcine coronary arteries. *J Vasc Surg.* 2004 Dec;40(6): 1216–22.

Shar BH, Nawaz Z. Inhibitory effect of curcumin, a food spice from turmeric, on platelet-activating factor- and arachidonic acid-mediated platelet aggregation through inhibition of thromboxane formation and Ca2+ signaling. *Biochem Pharmacol.* 1999 Oct 1;58(7):11 67–72.

Li HL, Liu C et al. Curcumin prevents and reverses murine cardiac hypertrophy. *J Clin Invest.* 2008 Feb 21.

Zhao J, Zhao Y et al. Neuroprotective effect of curcumin on transient focal cerebral ischemia in rats. *Brain Res.* 2008 Sep 10;1229:224–32. Epub 2008 Jul 8.

Chapter 3

Aggarwal BB, Kumar A et al. Anticancer potential of curcumin: preclinical and clinical studies. *Anticancer Res.* 2003 Jan–Feb;23(1A):363–398.

Link A, Balaquer F. Cancer chemoprevention by dietary polyphenols: promising role for epigenetics. *Biochem Pharmacol.* 2010 Dec 15;80(12):1771–92. Epub 2010 Jun 26.

Anand P, Sundaram C. Curcumin and cancer: an "old-age" disease with an "age-old" solution. *Cancer Lett.* 2008 Aug 18;267(1):133–164. Epub 2008 May 6.

Ireson CR, Jones DJ et al. Metabolism of the cancer chemopreventive agent curcumin in human and rat intestine. *Cancer Epidemiol Biomarkers Prev.* 2002; 11(1):105–111.

Cheng AL, Hsu CH et4 al. Phase I clinical trial of curcumin, a chemopreventive agent, in patients with high-risk or pre-malignant lesions. *Anticancer Res.* 2001;21(4B):2895–2900.

Nanji AA, Jokelainen K et al. Curcumin prevents alcohol-induced liver disease in rats by inhibiting the expression of NF-kappa B-dependent genes. *Am J Physiol Gastrointest Liver Physiol.* 2003 Feb;284(2):G321–7. Epub 2002 Aug 28.

Chapter 4

Chandran B, Goel A. A randomized study to assess the efficacy and safety of curcumin in patients with active rheumatoid arthritis. *Phytother Res.* March 9, 2012 doi: 10.1002/ptrr.4639.

Antony B, Kizhakedath et al. Clinical evaluation of a herbal product (Rhulief™) in the management of knee osteoarthritis. Abstract 316. *Osteoarthritis Cartilage.* 2011; 19(S1): S145-S146

Rao TS, Basu N et al. Anti-inflammatory activity of curcumin analogues. *Indian J Med Res.* 1982 Apr;75:574–578.

Funk JL, Ovarzo JN et al. Turmeric extracts containing curcuminoids prevent experimental rheumatoid arthritis. *J Nat Prod.* 2006 Mar;69(3):351–355.

Aggarwal BB, Sung B. Pharmacological basis for the role of curcumin in chronic diseases: an age-old spice with modern targets. *Trends Pharmacol Sci.* 2009; 30:85–94.

Liacini A, Sylvester J et al. Induction of matrix metalloproteinase-13 gene expression by TNF-alpha is mediated by MAP kinases, AP-1, and NF-kappaB transcription factors in articular chondrocytes. *J. Exp Cell Res.* 2003 Aug 1;288(1): 208–217.

Chapter 5

Fujiwara H, Hosokawa M et al. Curcumin inhibits glucose production in isolated mice hepatcytes. *Diabetes Res Clin Pract.* 2008 May;80(2):185–91. Epub 2008 Jan 24.

Weisberg SP, Leibel R et al. Dietary Curcumin Significantly Improves Obesity-Associated Inflammation and Diabetes in Mouse Models of Diabesity. *Endocrinology.* 2008 Jul;149(7):3549–58. Epub 2008 Apr 10.

Kulkarni SK, Chopra K. Curcumin the active principle of turmeric (Curcuma longa), ameliorates diabetic nephropathy in rats. *Clin Exp Pharmacol Physiol.* 2006 Oct;33(10): 940–945.

Chapter 6

Baum L et al. Six-month randomized placebo-controlled, double-blind, pilot clinical trial of curcumin in patients with Alzheimer's Disease. *Journal of Clinical Psychopharmacology.* Vol 28, Number 1, Feb 2008 pg 110–114

Xu Y, Ku B et al. Curcumin reverses impaired hippocampal neurogenesis and increases serotonin receptor 1A mRNA and brain-derived neurotrophic factor expression in chronically stressed rats. *Brain Res.* 2007 Aug 8;1162:9–18. Epub 2007 Jun 21.

Lim GP, Chu T et al. The curry spice curcumin reduces oxidative damage and amyloid pathology in an Alzheimer transgenic mouse. *J Neurosci.* 2001 Nov 1; 21(21):8370–77.

Garcia-Alloza M, Borrelli LA et al. Curcumin labels amyloid pathology in vivo, disrupts existing plaques, and partially restores distorted neurites in an Alzheimer mouse model, *J. Neurochem.* 102 (2007) 1095–1104.

Chapter 7

Sanmukhani J, Anovadiya A et al. Evaluation of antidepressant like activity of curcumin and its combination with fluoxetine and imipramine: an acute and chronic study. *Acta Pol Pharm.* 2011 Sep-Oct;68(5):769–75.

Baker CB. Quantitative Analysis of Sponsorship Bias in Economic Studies of Antidepressants. *The British Journal of Psychiatry.* 2003, 183: 498–506.

Kulkarni S, Dhir A et al. Potentials of curcumin as an antidepressant. *Scientific World-Journal.* 2009 Nov 1;9:1233–41.

Kulkarni S, Bhutani MK et al. Antidepressant activity of curcumin: involvement of serotonin and dopamine system. *Psychopharmacology (Berl).* 2008 Dec;201(3): 435–42. Epub 2008 Sep 3.

Chapter 8

Bundy R, et al. Turmeric extract may improve irritable bowel syndrome symptomology in otherwise healthy adults: a pilot study. *J Altern Complement Med.* 2004 Dec;10(6): 1015–18.

Kawamori T, et al. Chemopreventive effect of curcumin, a naturally occurring anti-inflammatory agent, during the promotion/progression stages of colon cancer. *Cancer Res.* 1999;59:597–601.

Chapter 9

Uysal KT, Wiesbrock SM et al. Protection from obesity-induced insulin resistance in mice lacking TNF-alpha function. *Nature.* 1997, 389:610–614.

Leray V, Freuchet B et al. Effect of citrus polyphenol and curcumin-supplemented diet on inflammatory state in obese cats. *Br J Nutr.* 2011 Oct;106 Suppl 1:S198–201.]

Lago F Dieguez C et al. Adipokines as emerging mediators of immune response and inflammation. *Nat Clin Pract Rhematoll.* 2007 3:716–724.

Awasthi S, Srivatava SK, Piper JT, Singhal SS, Chaubey M, Awasthi YC. Curcumin protects against 4-hydroxy-2-trans-nonenal-induced cataract formation in rat lenses. *Am J Clin Nutr.* 1996 Nov;64(5):761–766.

Rai D, Yadav D et al. Design and development of curcumin bioconjugates as antiviral agents. *Nucleic Acids Symp Ser (Oxf).* 2008;(52):599–600.

Bright JJ. Curcumin and autoimmune disease. *Adv Exp Med Biol.* 2007; 595: 425–451.

Chapter 10

Benny M, Antony B. Bioavailability of BioCurcumax™ (BCM-95®). *Spice India.* September, 2006:11–15.

Merina B, Iyer VS, et al. A pilot cross-over study to evaluate human oral bioavailability of BCM-95CG (Biocurcumax), a novel bioenhanced preparation of curcumin. *Ind J Pharm Sci.* 2008;70(4):445–449.

Poster presentation. Oral Bioavailability of BCM-95® Curcumin in Dogs. 2009 ACVIM Forum/Canadian VMA Convention: June 3–6, 2009; Montréal, Québec, Canada.]

Antony B, Merina B et al. A pilot cross-over study to evaluate human oral bioavailability of BCM-95® CG (Biocurcumax) a novel bioenhanced preparation of curcumin. *Ind J Pharm Sci.* 2008;70(4):445–450.

Bhardwaj R, Glaeser H et al. Piperine, a Major Constituent of Black Pepper, Inhibits Human P-glycoprotein and CYP3A4. *The Journal of Pharmacology and Experimental Therapeutics.* 2002 Aug;302(2):645–650.

Index

About the Author

Dr. Jan McBarron received her M.D. from Hahnemann University in Philadelphia and was the fourth woman in the country to become board certified in bariatric medicine. She is a member of the American Medical Association and the American Society of Bariatric Physicians. She volunteered with the 1996 Olympics, has been honored by the Girl Scouts as a "Woman of Achievement" and the Natural Products Association awarded her the "Clinician of the Year" for 2010.

While practicing bariatric and preventive medicine, Dr. McBarron became disenchanted with the mainstream allopathic medical system and its side effects. She subsequently earned a doctorate in naturopathic medicine and is one of the elite few to hold both medical and naturopathic degrees. She believes this enables her to see the complete picture and offer the best in complementary medicine.

Dr. McBarron taught at Columbus State University, writes for several newspapers and has appeared on numerous radio and television interviews. She is the author of several books including the best-selling *Flavor Without Fat, Being a Woman Naturally, Hormonal Harmony* and *The Peachtree Diet.*

In addition to her private medical practice, Georgia Bariatrics in Columbus, GA, Dr. McBarron co-hosts the #1 nationally syndicated health talk radio show "Duke and The Doctor," with her husband, Duke Liberatore. *Talkers Magazine* has ranked them in the top 100 most important radio hosts in America. They are broadcast in over 125 markets nationwide. For a list of their radio station affiliates visit www.dukeandthedoctor.com.